Once a Fitness for Men

A Fitness Programme for Men of All Ages

by

Barbara Roberton

PSL

Patrick Stephens
Wellingborough, Northamptonshire

First published February 1987

© BARBARA ROBERTON 1987

British Library Cataloguing in Publication Data

Roberton, Barbara
Once a week fitness for men: a fitness
programme for men of all ages.
1. Exercise for men   2. Physical fitness for men
I. Title
613.7'1 088041   RA781

ISBN 1-85260-0004

*Patrick Stephens Limited is part of the
Thorsons Publishing Group,
Wellingborough, Northamptonshire, NN8 2RQ, England.*

Printed in Great Britain by
Woolnough Bookbinding Limited,
Irthlingborough, Northamptonshire

5   7   9   10   8   6

*Dedicated to Alan, Nicola, Katy,
and Dizzy*

Contents

Introduction

Once a Week Fitness is for men of all ages, shapes and sizes. It aims to explore the different ways that men can exercise and will help you find the one most suited to you, your lifestyle and, most importantly, the one you most enjoy.

The way a man looks and holds himself says a lot about the way he feels and how he looks after his body. Eating sensibly and exercising at least *once a week* will trim your figure, give you added stamina and generally improve your attitude to life.

This book is to help tone up your muscles, firm up any 'flab' and develop a positive mental attitude.

How to Start

Take a good look at yourself, think about your present lifestyle–

Are you overweight?
Do you drink a lot of beer?
Do you drive everywhere and not take regular exercise?
Do you yawn and feel drowsy all afternoon?
Are you too tired to play with the kids?
Do you ever say 'I'm getting old?' – You are – but don't let it happen too soon.

Now is the time to start, you need determination, a little will power and the desire to get fit and stay fit.

What Kind of Exercise

There are many ways of exercising. You can exercise alone by running, walking cycling or swimming or you can participate in a team with football training or a Rugby Club. There are also many facilities available at your local gym. You must decide which suits you best and which you most enjoy. The exercises in this book are muscle toning exercises based on my many years experience as a dancer and teacher of dance and keep fit. They are designed to make you aware of yourself and your body.

Benefits of Exercise

By following the programme with determination and will power, and of course a sensible diet you will soon find:

- your stomach and chest are firmer
- your posture more upright
- you have increased stamina and vitality
- you will also feel generally healthier and happier.

Think Fit

Your attitude towards yourself is *very important*. Have a positive attitude and it will show in the way you stand and walk. It will also show in your face, and enable you to project a good image. After all the first thing others notice is the way you look. First impressions last. However, we want to go deeper than that. The man that takes good care of his body is more likely to take good care of his mind; the way he tackles things at work and his attitude in all sorts of situations. You are your own best friend or your own worst enemy. Life is very short. Enjoy life, think fit, healthy and happy. Don't let petty irritations get you down. Once you make this committment you are on your way to a vibrant and joyous lifestyle.

The workings of the mind and body are intriguing. Study suggests that exercise produces both physical and psychological changes which enhance the quality of life and improves our abilities to think and act.

Make Time to Exercise

Get into the habit of exercise. Make it part of your life, like eating and sleeping. *You owe it to your body* to stay young and fit whatever your age. Use everyday tasks as a form of exercise. Always exercise with care, especially if you are embarking on it for the first time, or after a long lapse of time.

Diet

The basics of life are food, drink and sleep – most men have too little sleep and far too much of the other two. Expense account lunches, putting the world to right over a pint, too much sugar and the list goes on. We must understand that the food we consume is fuel to the body, any excess will turn to fat. Stop and think before taking another potato, one more pint of beer or a second spoonful of sugar in your tea.

Educate your stomach to expect less food and it will soon respond. Drink more water – carbonated mineral waters are really enjoyable and will work wonders for your kidneys.

Stress – and Learning to Relax

Stress and tension can cause many problems for the man of today. Time is so short and everything has to be done in such a hurry. Exercise can take away a lot of the feelings of tension and stress. Stress can bring on so many symptoms – aches and pains, headaches, raised blood-pressure and at worst angina and heart attacks. Don't let it happen to you. Documented risk factors for heart disease include; family history, being overweight, high blood-pressure, high intake of animal fats – not enough exercise and stress. The art of relaxation has to be learnt and practised. Give yourself a few minutes each day to unwind and slow down. It will ease your headaches, and take the tightness out of your neck, shoulders and chest. It will greatly improve your temper and you will be a much nicer person to know.

Always relax after exercising – use the time to slow down your heart and pulse rate. The worked muscles can cool slowly and thus prevent cramps and strains.

What to Wear

Be comfortable – never exercise in tight clothing, be unrestricted and warm. Muscles need to be kept warm in order to prevent injury. Shoes should be well fitting and secure. Always remove any jewellery, nasty accidents can be caused by loose rings, neck chains and the like.

Pain

If it hurts – STOP! The golden rule is never strain. There are two different types of pain. There is the stiffness we get if we exercise too vigorously, having done very little for a long time – it is temporary – take a warm bath and it will soon pass. Then there is injury pain which is sharp and stabbing. Injury pain should always be investigated. Don't make unreasonable demands on your body. Start slowly and gently build up to a level you can maintain. You can then work to constantly improve as you see and feel the results.

Before Exercising

Always make sure you have an empty bladder. Don't eat a heavy meal or drink alcohol as this may result in cramp or nausea.

Check List

If you have any heart condition, hypertension or serious varicose veins you should consult your doctor as to the level of exercise he considers sensible for you. Listen to your body – if anything hurts STOP. Pay special attention to exercises involving your back. Start gently and build up gradually, NEVER STRAIN.

Exercising should be fun as well as beneficial. Make sure you enjoy what you are doing and you will soon enjoy the results.

How to use this book

Many forms of exercise are explored and it is up to you to experiment and to find the one most suited to you. These exercises are designed to tone you up, and make you more supple. When put together they will take one hour. The box in the corner of each page is the ideal number of repetitions or length of time to aim for. Make this your goal. They can be done with or without music, whichever you prefer. Music does add to the enjoyment, a cassette tape is a good idea, it saves you changing records.

Start slowly and carefully and work your way up to the ideal. Always remember not to strain, start gently and if it hurts – STOP.

Running and Jogging

You're never too fat, too old or too slow to start running. Running is marvellous all-round exercise, improving the capacity of your heart and lungs. It is probably the easiest form of exercise. All you need is a track suit and a good pair of well fitting shoes and a stop watch. Incorrect footwear will certainly harm your ankles or knees and may cause back injury. So it is essential to have the right shoes. A sports shop will advise you.

Build up slowly, starting with brisk walking;

increase your speed and distance at your own pace. Time yourself and keep a record of your progress. It has been said that jogging is boring but many athletes in the peak of condition experience 'runners' high' where they feel their minds are disassociated from their bodies. On the way to reaching such heights enjoy running with a friend, look at the trees and birds and experience the clean air – ENJOY IT.

Sport

Sports such as golf and bowling are unlikely to be of much value because of the long pauses in such games. Continuous movement is what is needed such as basketball, squash, skating, skiing and hiking. Tennis depends on the quality and speed of play. Brisk walking is ideal for those in poor physical condition and the elderly.

Swimming is an ideal, all round exercise.

Weight training can be of considerable benefit. High repetitions with weights will increase stamina and muscle power. There are a variety of exercise machines available in well equipped clubs and centres.

Team sports Football and rugby require a high degree of fitness and speed but not necessarily suppleness. Training consists of a great deal of running and sprinting, press ups, squat thrusts, and sit ups, and of course catching, tackling and dribbling with the ball.

Basketball is one of the fastest of indoor games. It is often used as a training exercise for many different sports and makes an ideal conclusion to circuit training.

Which ever type of exercise you choose – enjoy it – it is no good doing something you hate, The more you enjoy what you are doing the greater the benefits. You owe it to your body to get fit and keep fit.

Warm-up

(1) **(2)**

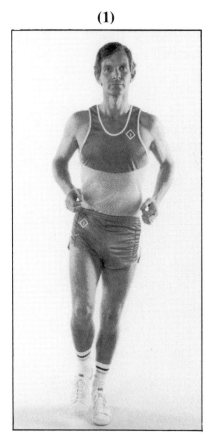 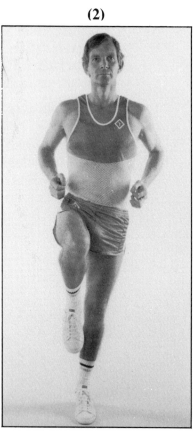

Before exercising it is essential that your muscles are well warmed up, in order to prevent strains and pulls. Start by walking, with your tummy pulled in tight and your shoulders back. Now jog on the spot for about two minutes **(1)**. Lift the knees higher and continue for a further two minutes **(2)**.

WARM UP	IDEAL
JOG	2 MINS
KNEES UP	2 MINS
JUMPS	12
BOUNCE	12

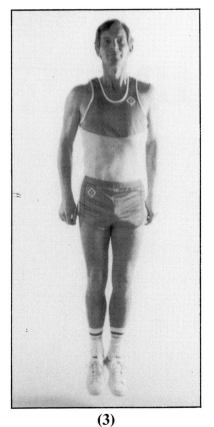

(3)

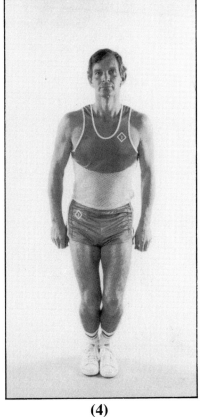

(4)

Jump on the spot as high as you can for as long as you can in comfort (3). They gently bounce in place till you feel really warm (4).

Toe Touching

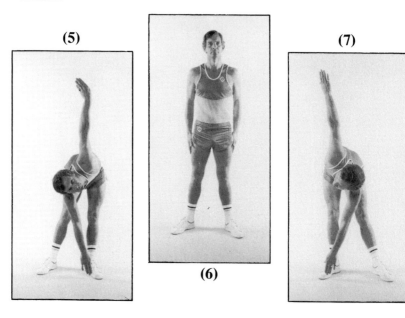

(5)

(6)

(7)

For suppleness

Stand with your feet apart and take the right hand over to the left foot **(5)** then straighten up **(6)**. Take the left hand to the right foot **(7)**, straighten the back **(6)**. Place both hands on the floor between your legs and push forward three times **(8)** – stretch up. Make the three movements flow freely and rhythmically.

	IDEAL
TOE TOUCHES	**20**
SWINGS	**20**

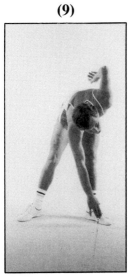

(9)

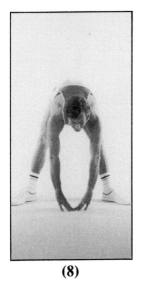

(8)

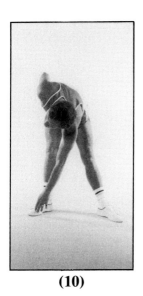

(10)

You will find it easier to slightly bend your knees to start with. Now swing from side to side, touching the inside of your ankle **(9) (10)**.

Bending

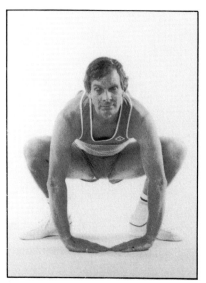

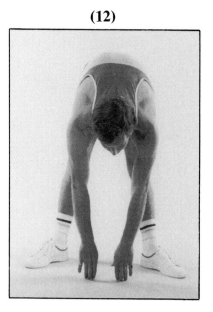

(12)

(11)

Feet apart, fold in half, hands on the floor and bend your knees **(11)**. Push your bottom up and straighten your knees **(12)**. Push up and down gently, don't strain, if your back hurts – STOP.

	IDEAL
BENDS FEET APART	**12**
BENDS FEET TOGETHER	**12**

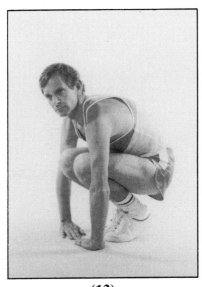

(13)

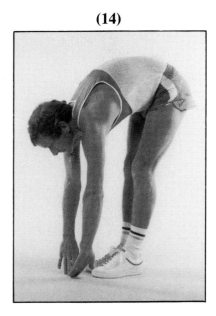

(14)

Place feet together, crouch down and hold your ankles **(13)**. Stretch up and straighten legs **(14)**. Keep stretching, making sure you straighten your legs.

Stand up and have a wriggle, shake out the legs to prevent any stiffness.

Jumps

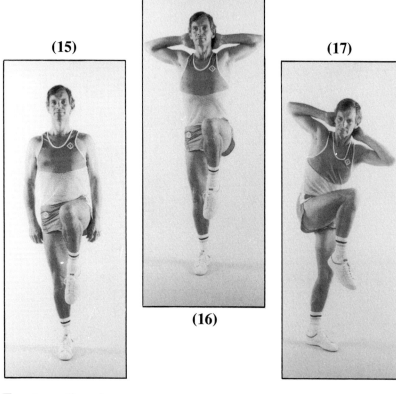

(15)

(16)

(17)

To strengthen legs

On the spot, jump and bring your knees up as high as is comfortable **(15)** one leg then the other. Then with the hands behind your head **(16)**.

Without jumping, lift knee to opposite elbow **(17)**.

	IDEAL
KNEES UP	48
HANDS BEHIND HEAD	48
KNEE TO ELBOW	24

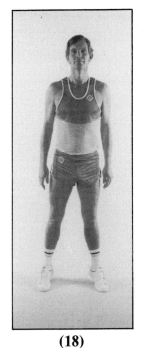

(18)

(19)

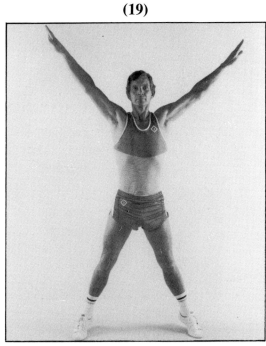

Jump feet apart **(18)** and back together four times − then jump feet apart taking arms up to form an 'X' **(19)**. Make this bouncy and rhythmic, four without arms, four with arms. Keep going for as long as you can.

	IDEAL
JUMPS	24
WITH ARMS	24
APART/TOGETHER	24
CONTINUOUS	24

(20)

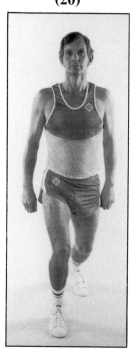

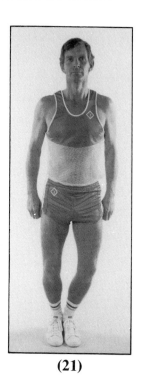

(22)

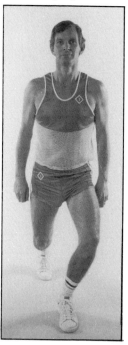

(21)

Jump feet apart right foot forward, knees bent **(20)** now jump feet together again **(21)**. Then jump left foot forward **(22)** and back together again.

Now try jumping foot to foot and keep going.

Waist

	IDEAL
WAIST PUSHES	**24**
HANDS ON HIPS	**24**
BEHIND HEAD	**24**

Trimmer

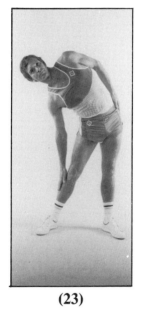
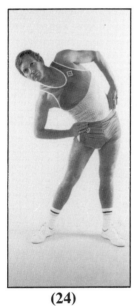
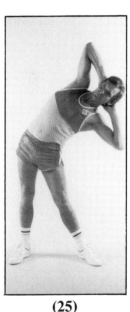

(23)	(24)	(25)

Lose inches

Feet apart and push from the waist, sliding your hand down your leg towards the knee **(23)**. Four to one side, four to the other side, then eight pushes side to side.

Place your hands on your hips and rock from side to side **(24)**.

Place your hands behind your head and rock from side to side **(25)**. Keep going and see the results.

Arm Swings

(26) **(27)**

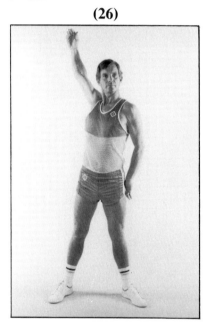 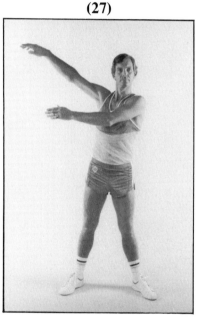

For arms and chest

Stand up straight, feet apart and circle right arm backwards three times **(26)**, then circle the left arm backwards three times. Swing both arms around in front of the body three times in one direction, then three times in the other direction **(27)**.

	IDEAL
ARM SWINGS	**12**
ARM FLINGS	**12**

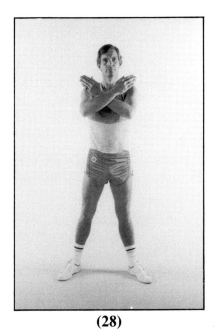

(28)

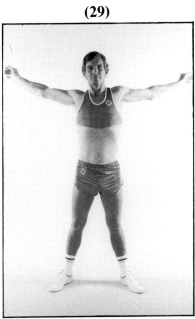

(29)

Bring arms in to cross the chest **(28)**. Fling the arms back **(29)** then back to **(28)**. You will feel this pull across the chest and the upper arm.

Floor Work

Lie down on a mat or a thick towel; not only does this cushion your back, it also stops you sliding about, especially if you are on a polished floor. For a few seconds lie flat and relax. Let everything go!

Try to tighten each of your muscles separately. Work through your calves, thighs, and tummy. Then really pull in your buttocks. Then let them go.

Remember, DON'T STRAIN. Do all the exercises at your own pace – build up gradually. All sit ups should be done through a curved spine, if it hurts – STOP.

However, don't be lazy. Make your body work.

Sit Ups and Stretches

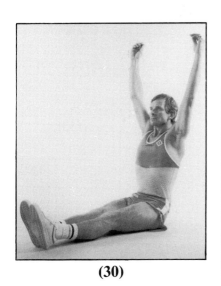

(30)

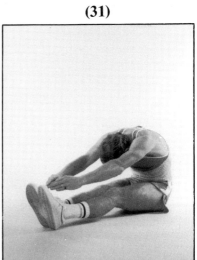

(31)

Abdominal strengthener

Lie flat on the floor, and pull stomach in, sit up, reach up
with your hands, diaphragm lifted and tummy tight **(30)**.
Fold as flat as you can **(31)**. With all sit ups come up and go
down through a curved spine to avoid hurting your back.

	IDEAL
SIT UPS **of each variation**	**10**

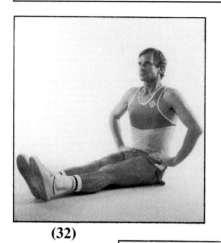

(32)

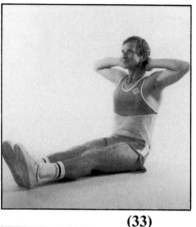

(33)

(33a)

Place your hands on your hips and sit up straightening the spine **(32)**. Then put your hands behind your head and sit up. Keep your elbows well back and don't pull on your neck **(33)**.

When you can do the above sit ups comfortably, try doing them with your knees bent and feet flat on the floor **(33a)**.

	IDEAL
ELBOW TO KNEE	**10**
HAND TO TOE	**10**

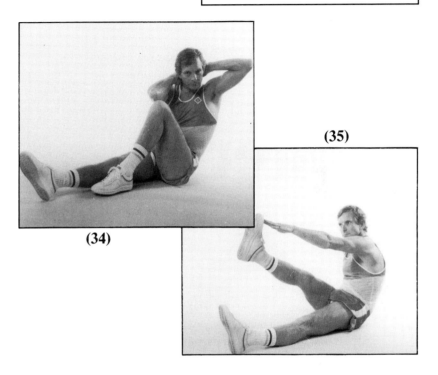

(34)

(35)

Lie flat, put your hands behind your head. Sit up and at the same time bring the opposite knee up to touch your elbow **(34)**. Lie back down again and sit up to the other side.

Lie flat, sit up and at the same time lift the right leg and touch foot with your left hand **(35)**. Lie down again, then repeat on the other side.

You may find these hard to start with, if so try them both from a sitting position. Gradually you will feel it getting easier.

Thigh and Tummy Toner

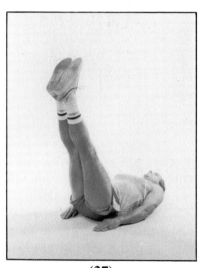

(37)

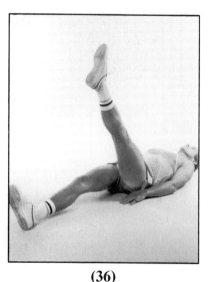

(36)

	IDEAL
LEG LIFTS	6 SETS
HANDS BEHIND HEAD	6 SETS
HANDS ON MIDRIFF	6 SETS

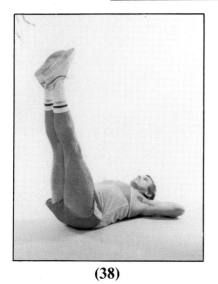

(38)

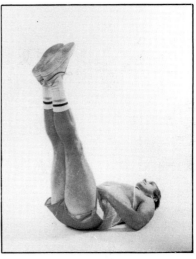

(38a)

Firm up any 'flab'

Lie flat, tummy pulled in. Lift one leg, slowly, and lower it, then the other **(36)**. Now lift both legs together, lower and lift them up again **(37)**. Make your tummy do the work, control the legs, don't let them crash to the floor.

Try the same exercise with your hands behind your head **(38)**. The place your hands on your midriff and repeat the exercise **(38a)**.

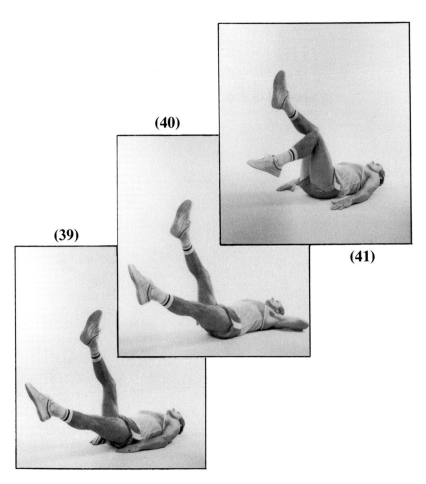

(40)

(39)

(41)

Lie flat, hands cushioning your back. Lift one leg up, and change legs in mid air **(39)**. Try to keep your legs straight and your toes pointed. Start with just a few and work your way up to the ideal.

When you can do this easily, try putting your hands under your head **(40)**.

Lie flat, hands cushioning the base of your spine. Lift legs off the floor and cycle **(41)**. Keep going for as long as you can.

	IDEAL
LEG CHANGES	50
HANDS BEHIND HEAD	20
CYCLING	50
HANDS BEHIND HEAD	20
ELBOW TO KNEE	20

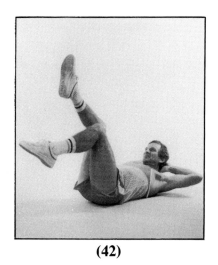

(42)

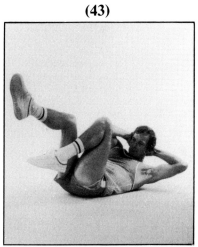

(43)

Next try cycling with your hands behind your head, and lift the shoulders slightly off the floor **(42)**.

When you can happily cycle with your hands behind your head, try taking your opposite elbow to your knee **(43)**. Keep your tummy pulled in. It is difficult but it gets easier the more you do it. But don't strain.

Thigh Strengthener

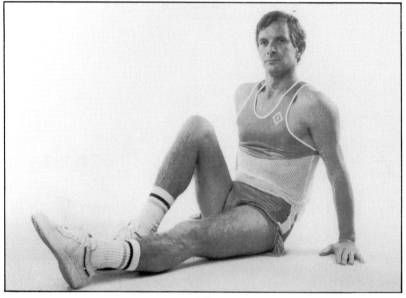

(44)

Upper thigh toner

Sit up straight, legs stretched out in front, toes pointed. Bring one knee up at a time, making sure to keep your back straight **(44)**. Do this twenty times slowly and then twenty times as quickly as you can. Keep your weight well forward off the base of your spine.

	IDEAL
LEG CHANGES	40
BOTH KNEES	20
HANDS BEHIND HEAD	20

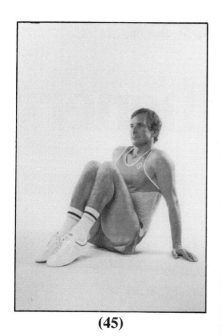

(45)

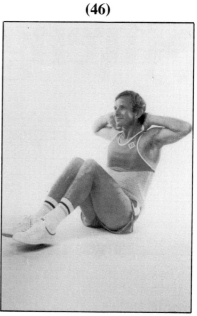

(46)

Now bring both knees up together and then stretch them out
(45). Keep your weight well forward and keep going for as
long as you can. Then do the same exercise with your hands
behind your head (46).

Relax and have a good wriggle to release any tension in the
legs.

Back and Shoulder Strengtheners

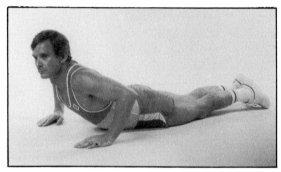

(47)

Gentle pushes

Roll onto your stomach and gently push up with your hands from the waist. Keep your shoulders down and your elbows tucked in. Work up to twelve pushes **(47)**.

Now push yourself up onto your knees **(48)** and all the way back into a tucked position **(49)** keeping the arms well in front. Push forward and return to the floor **(50)**.

	IDEAL
PUSH UPS	**12**
PUSHES INTO	
TUCKED POSITION	**12**

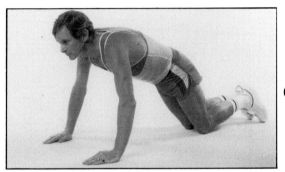

(48)

(49)

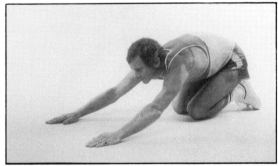

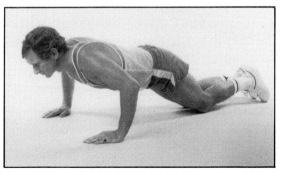

(50)

	IDEAL
PUSH UPS	**30**
BODY LIFT	**10**

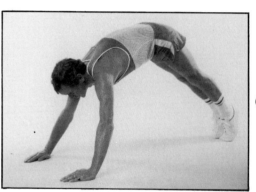

(51)

(52)

Lie flat and tuck your toes under. Push up on the hands until your arms are straight **(51)** lower to the ground. Do as many as is comfortable, building up gradually.

When you can do this well try lifting your body up **(52)** hold it for five counts then lower to the floor.

Always have a wriggle after these exercises to release the tightness.

Leg

	IDEAL
TOE TOUCHES	16
2 HANDS TO	
EACH FOOT	16
FOLD IN HALF	16

Stretches

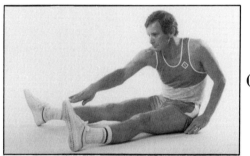

(53)

(54)

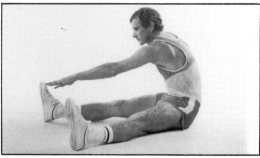

Inner thighs

Sit upright, back straight, feet apart as wide as you can. Take your right hand over to your left foot **(53)** then the left hand over to the right foot **(54)**. Then fold in half and push forward three times **(55)**. Pull up and straighten your back.

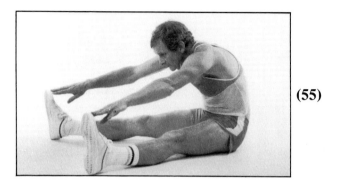

(55)

(56)

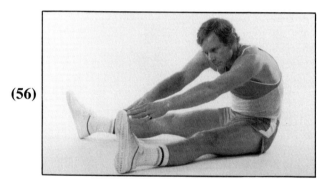

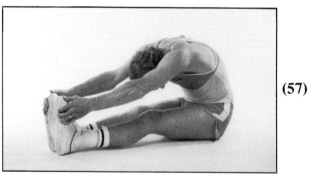

(57)

Now try taking both hands over to each foot **(56)**.

Then bring your feet together, sit up straight and fold in half, keeping your tummy well pulled in and your diaphragm lifted **(57)**.

Hamstring Stretch

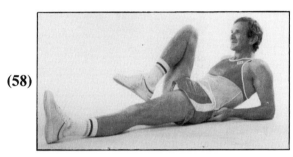

(58)

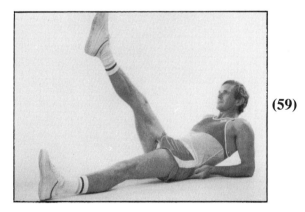

(59)

Back of legs

Sit up, lean back onto your elbows. Bring your knee in towards your chest **(58)**. Put it down then throw the same leg up straight **(59)**. First on one leg, then on the other.

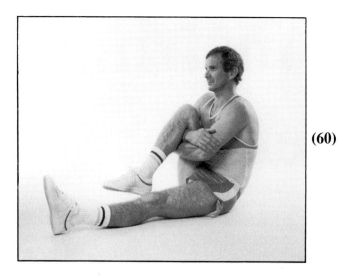

(60)

(61)

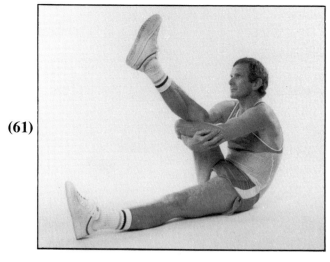

Next sit up straight and take hold of your leg underneath the knee **(60)**. Gently extend the leg, pointing your toes **(61)**. Work up to do ten stretches on each leg. Once the legs will stretch easily try rotating your feet in both directions and up and down. Now try both legs together **(62)** keeping your weight forward and off the base of the spine **(63)**.

	IDEAL
HAMSTRING STRETCH	**12 ON EACH LEG**
LEG FLEXES	**10 ON EACH LEG**
BOTH LEGS	**5**

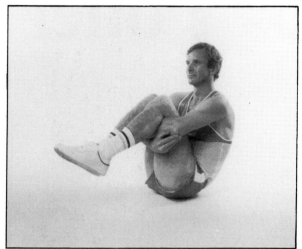

(62)

(63)

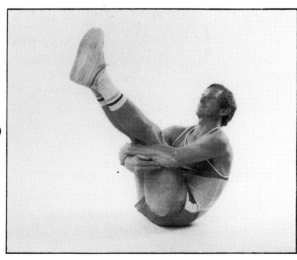

Thigh and Hip Toner

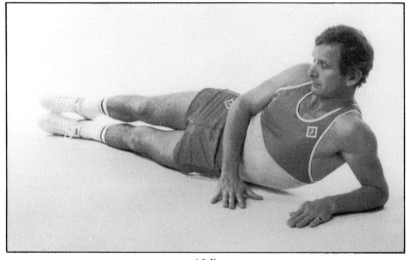

(64)

Hips and upper thigh

Lie on your side, keeping your hips well forward **(64)**. Throw your leg up **(65)**. Keep going for as long as you can, then repeat on the other side.

	IDEAL
LEG LIFTS	50
KNEES UP	20

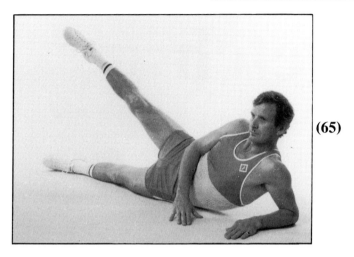

(65)

(66)

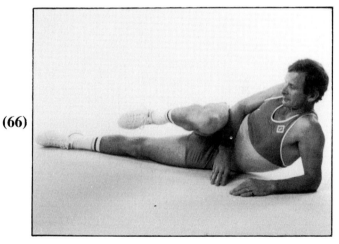

Then bend the knee and bring it up towards your face **(66)**.
Try ten on one side and then ten on the other.

Upward Stretch

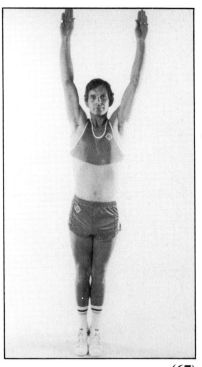

(67)

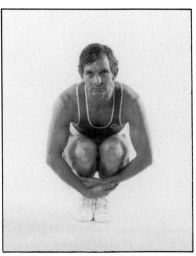

(68)

	IDEAL
PULL UPS	20
SWINGS	16
CLIMBS	30

All over stretch

Pull up onto your toes and stretch your abdomen. Reach up with your hands **(67)**. Bend the knees and crouch down into a tucked position **(68)**. Continue up and down.

Swing your arms and body in a circle from the waist, letting your hands touch the floor as you go round **(69, 70, 71, 72)**. First in one direction and then in the other.

Now climb up an imaginary rope above your head.

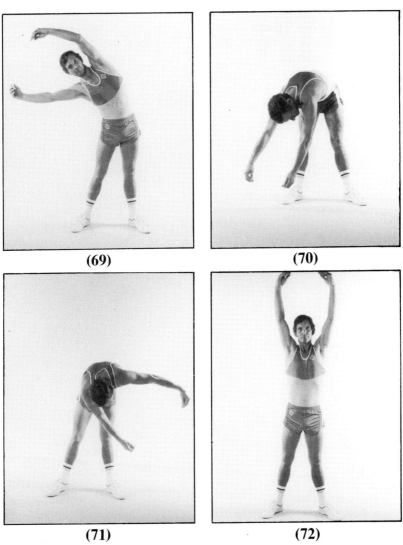

(69)

(70)

(71)

(72)

Forward Lunges

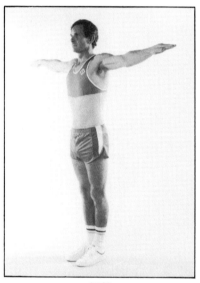

(73)

(74)

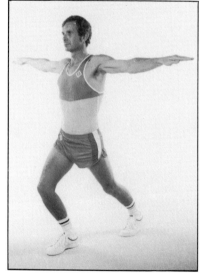

	IDEAL
LUNGES	10 ON EACH LEG
BOUNCES	10 ON EACH LEG
TRANSFERING WEIGHT	10 ON EACH LEG

(75)

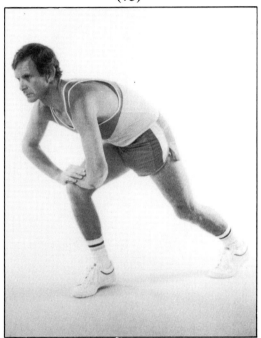

Thighs, hips and waist

Stand up straight, arms outstretched **(73)** take a forward lunge with the right foot **(74)**. Step back feet together again. Make ten lunges on the right leg then ten lunges with the left leg.

Take lunged position and gently bounce on bent leg **(75)**. Now the other leg.

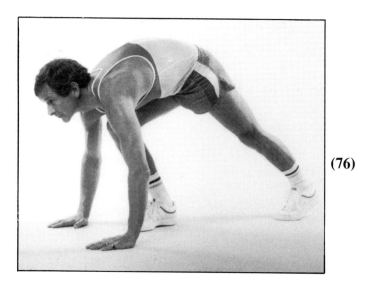

(76)

(77)

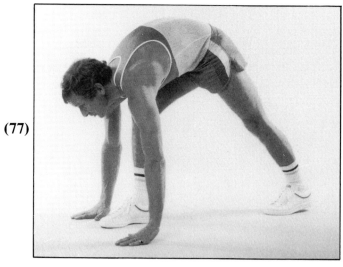

Take lunged position, lean forward and put the palms of your hands on the floor **(76)**. Transfer the weight from the front leg onto both feet straightening your legs **(77)**. Push forward and back five times. Then try on the other leg.

Leg Stretch

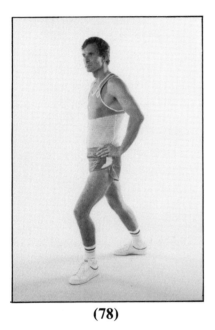

(78)

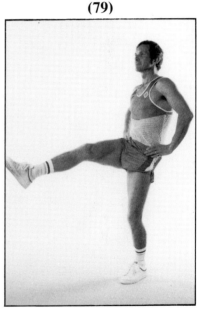

(79)

Upper leg toner

Stand up straight, step behind with right leg, allowing your supporting leg to bend **(78)**. Kick right leg up in front at the same time straightening supporting leg **(79)** and down again. Ten kicks on one leg and then ten kicks on the other leg.

	IDEAL
KICKS	**10**
KNEES	**10**

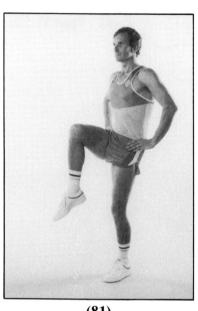

(81)

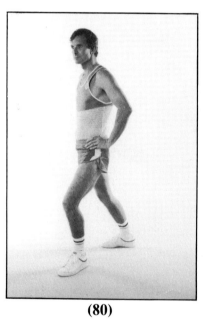

(80)

Now try the same exercise with working leg bent **(80) (81)**.

Knee Bends

	IDEAL
KNEE BENDS	**20**

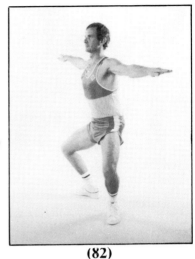
(82)

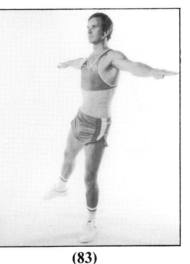
(83)

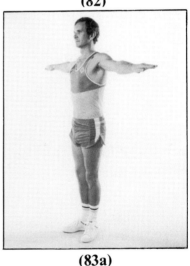
(83a)

Upper leg toner

Stand up straight, step right foot out to the side and bend both knees **(82)**. Lift up left leg and bring feet together **(83 and 83a)**.

Then step the left foot out to the side bending both knees. Lift up the right leg and bring feet together.

Waist Turns

	IDEAL
WAIST TURNS	50
DOUBLE PUSH	30
HANDS ON HIPS	50

(84)

(85)

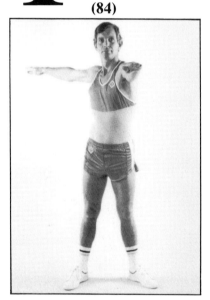

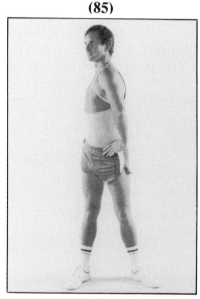

Lose inches

Stand up straight, feet apart and arms at shoulder height at a 90° angle **(84)**. Make sure you keep your hips and knees still and turn from the waist at least twenty times. Then make a double push to each side.

Place your hands on your hips, feet apart. Keep your hips and knees still and turn from the waist **(85)**.

Pull Ups

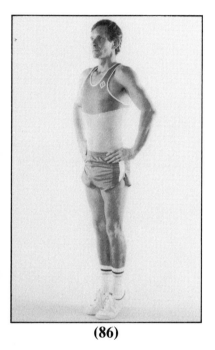

(86)

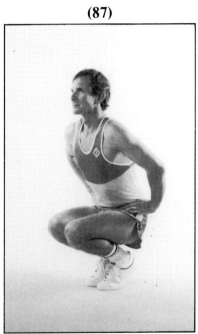

(87)

All over stretch

Stand up straight, hands on hips. Pull up onto toes **(86)**.
Bend the knees and down into a tucked position **(87)**. Up
again onto toes **(88)** lower heels **(89)**. Repeat five times to
start with and build up slowly.

	IDEAL
PULL UPS	**10**
WITH JUMP	**5**

(88)

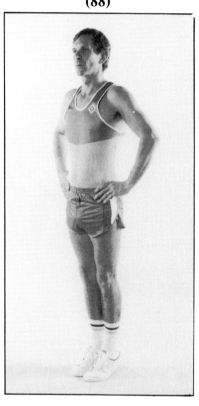

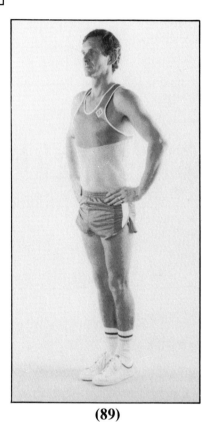

(89)

When you can do it comfortably, try jumping up from the tucked position. You will find it difficult to start with – but it will get easier.

Exercising With a Chair

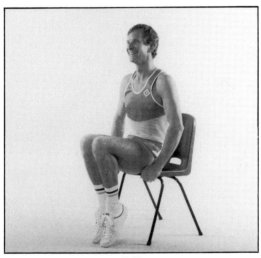

(90)

TUMMY TONER

Sit on the edge of an upright chair. Back straight and hold on to the edge **(90)**. Draw up your knees **(91)**. Extend the legs and hold for five counts, keeping your stomach pulled in tight **(92)**.

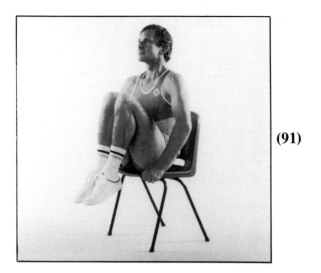

(91)

(92)

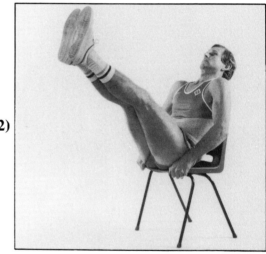

THIGH TIGHTENER

Sit upright on the chair. Lift the right leg and touch your toe
with your left hand **(93)**. Then touch the left toe with the right
hand. Keep touching opposite toe for as long as you can.

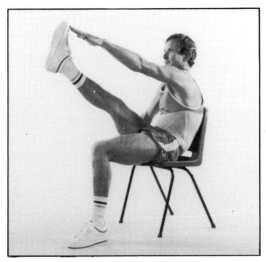

(93)

(94)

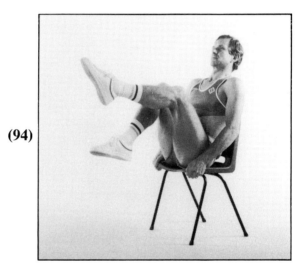

Now try holding on to the chair, lift your legs off the floor and cycle for as long as you can **(94)**.

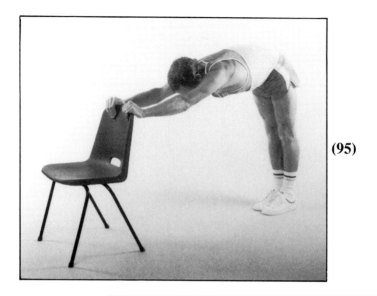

(95)

(96)

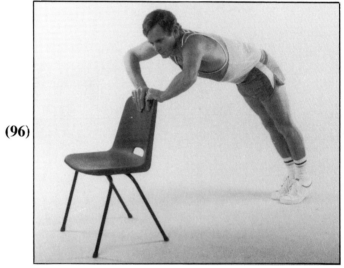

Stand up and hold on to the back of the chair **(95)**. Without bending the legs, push forward and allow the elbows to bend **(96)**.

Cool
Down

COOL DOWN
3–5 MINS
IDEAL

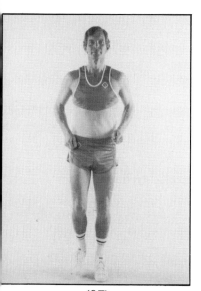

(97)

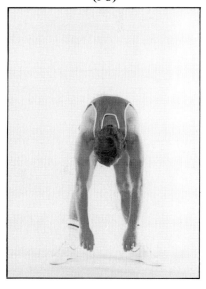

(98)

Cooling down is just as important as warming up. It allows the heart and pulse rates to slow down gradually and releases any tension in the worked muscles.

Jog on the spot for two minutes **(97)**. Then walk keeping shoulders back, tummy pulled in and swing legs from your hips and finally flop **(98)**.

Relaxation

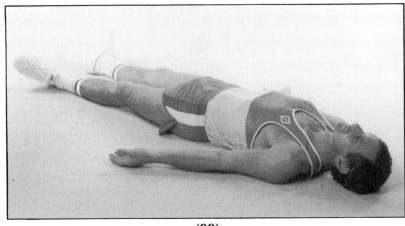

(99)

This is so important, after any exercise give your body time to slow down and cool down. Time spent in relaxation will enable you to tackle the rest of the day in a calm and happy way.

LIE DOWN, having first put on a warm sweater or track suit and some relaxing music. A lovely piece is Gymnopodie 1 and 3 by Erik Satie. Make yourself comfortable, feel all the tensions release. Start at your toes and work your way through all your limbs **(99)**.

Breath in through your nose and out through your mouth. Close your eyes and let yourself float away. Stay there for about five minutes or until the music stops. Then have a good wriggle and sit up when you are ready. You will feel wonderful, rested, calm and ready to tackle the rest of the day.